THE MARVELOUS STORY OF JESSICA AND THE STUPID BAD THING
A <u>Not for Kids</u> Tragedy

By Jessica

Published by Not for Kids Books
Story, characters, and illustrations
Copyright © 2016 Not for Kids Books
ISBN: 978-1530127832

To all the moms and dads that try so hard every day to get it right, without a manual, you're great!

Once upon a time,
in a city just like yours
and in a home
just like yours,
there lived
a wonderful couple.

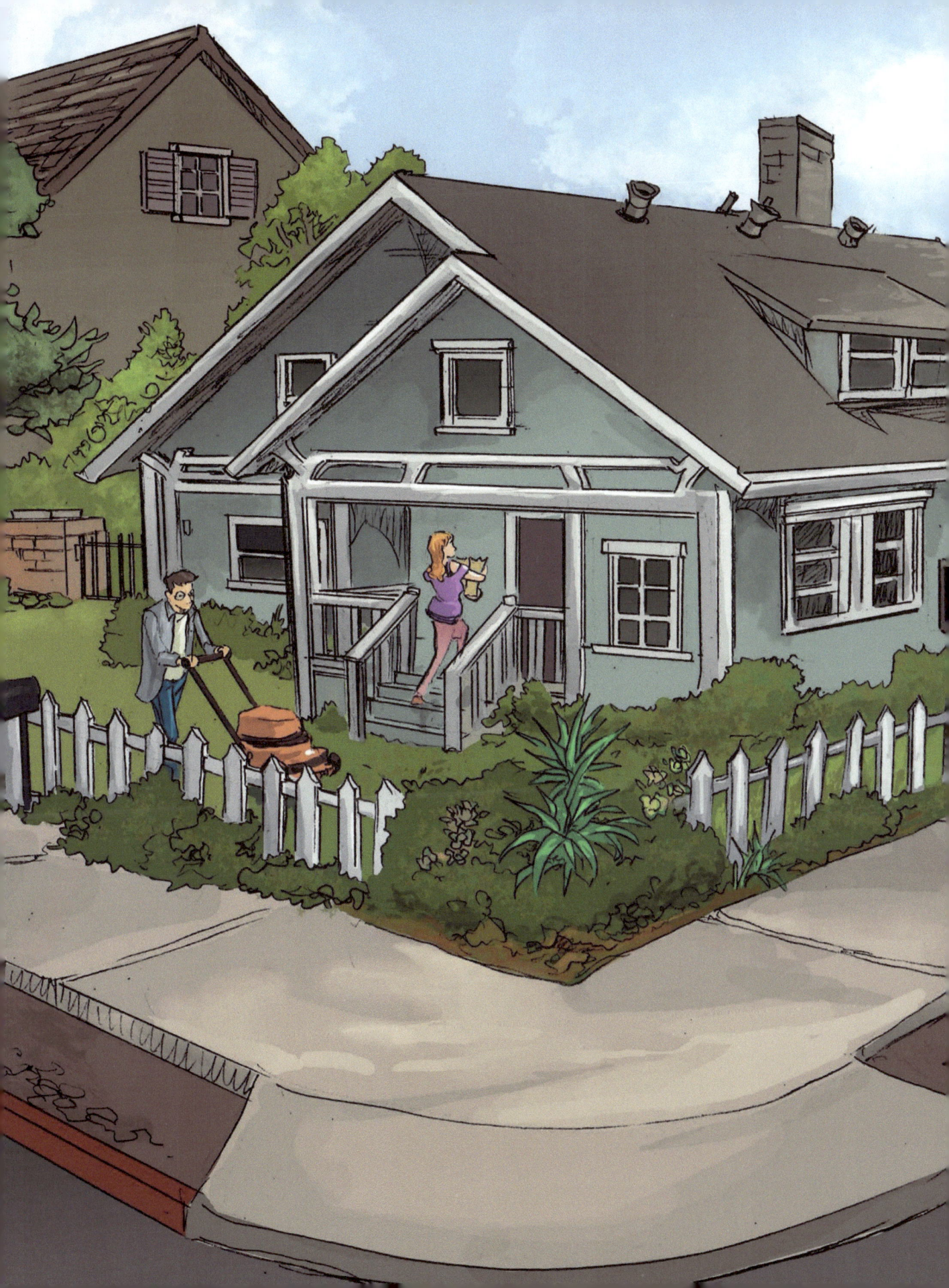

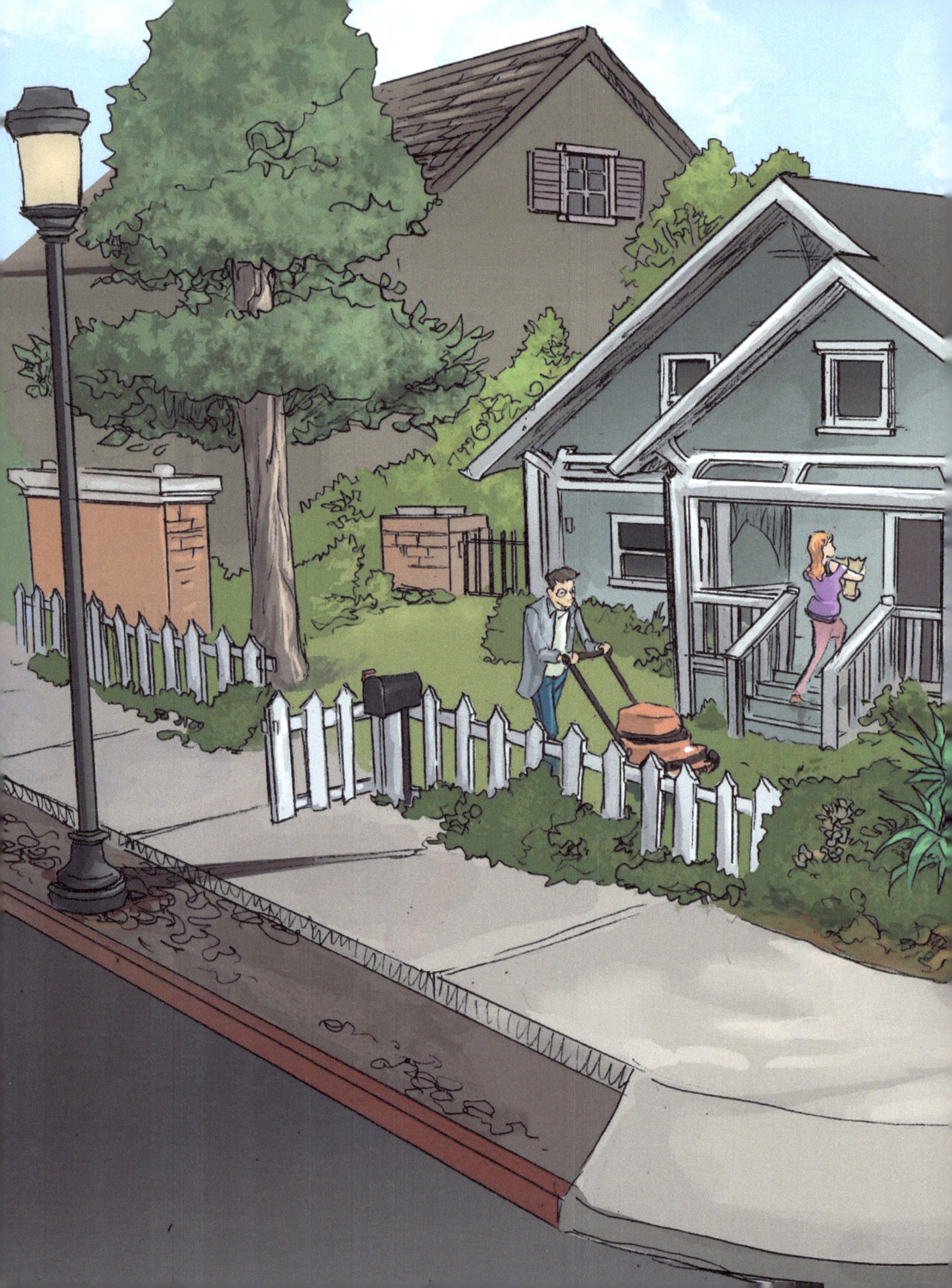

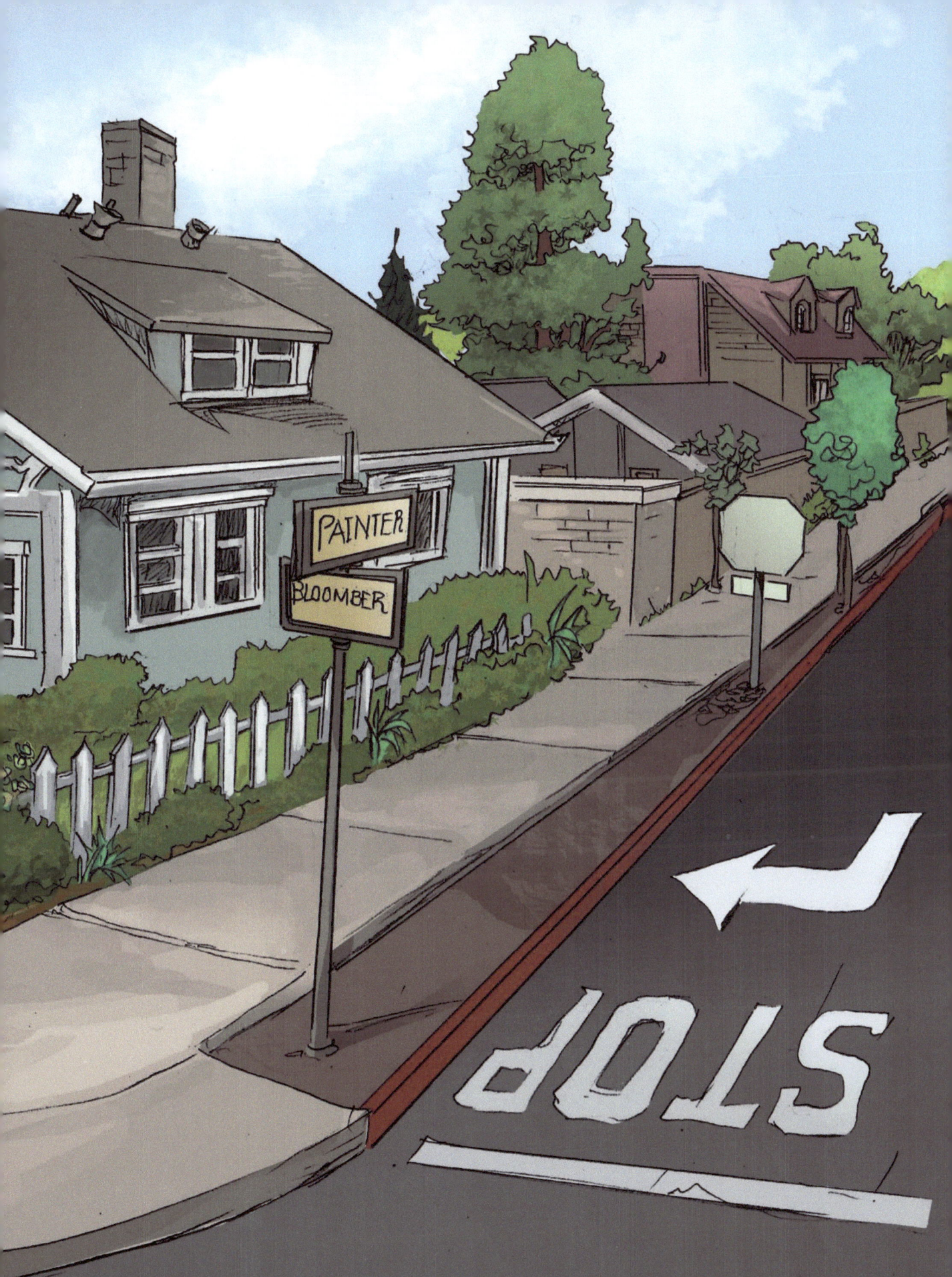

This wonderful couple was getting ready for the birth of their first child – a healthy baby girl. They decided to name her Jessica, and they made lots of plans for her future.

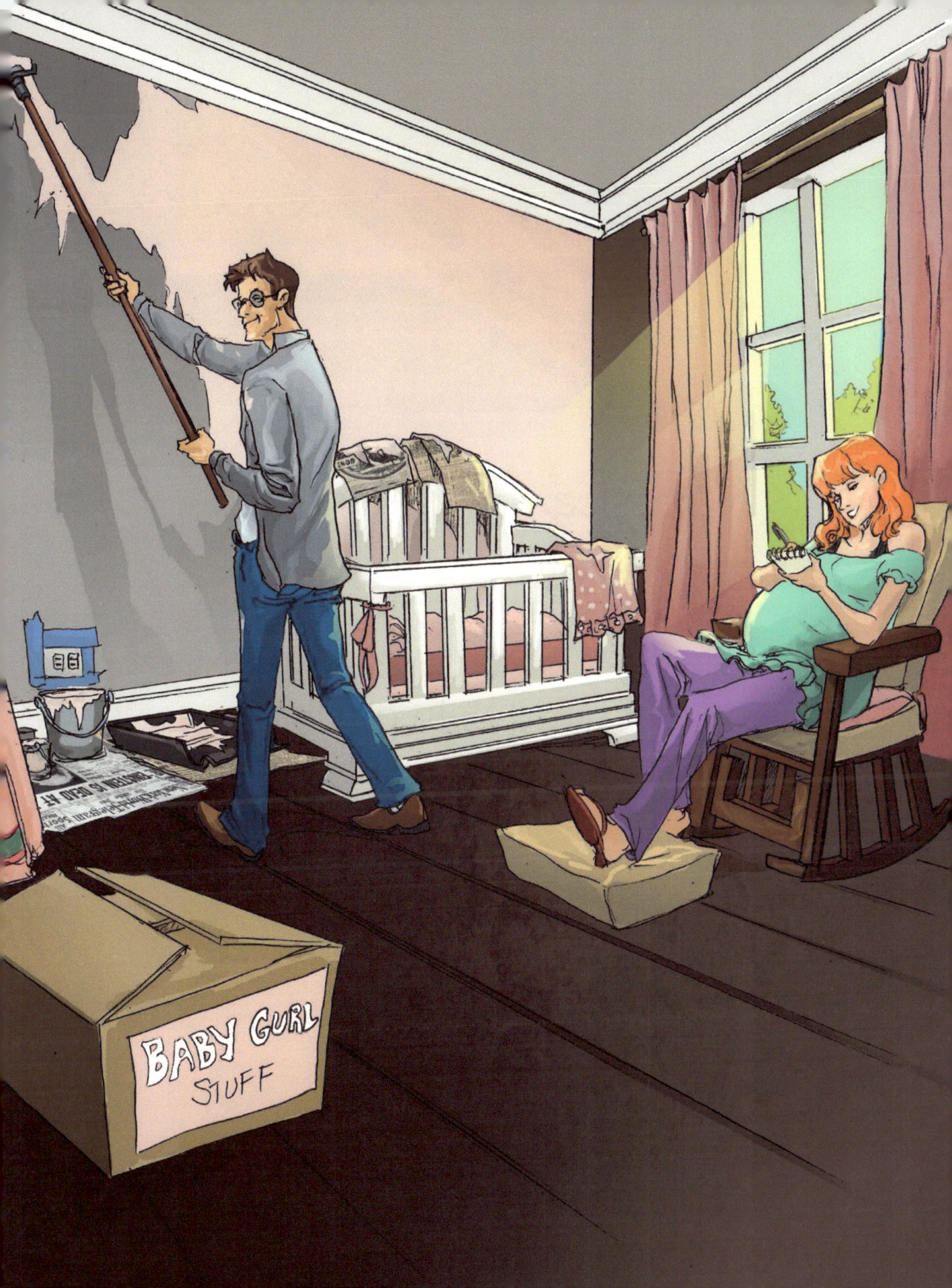

Jessica was born not too early and not too late. She came practically right on time, but she needed help coming into the world.

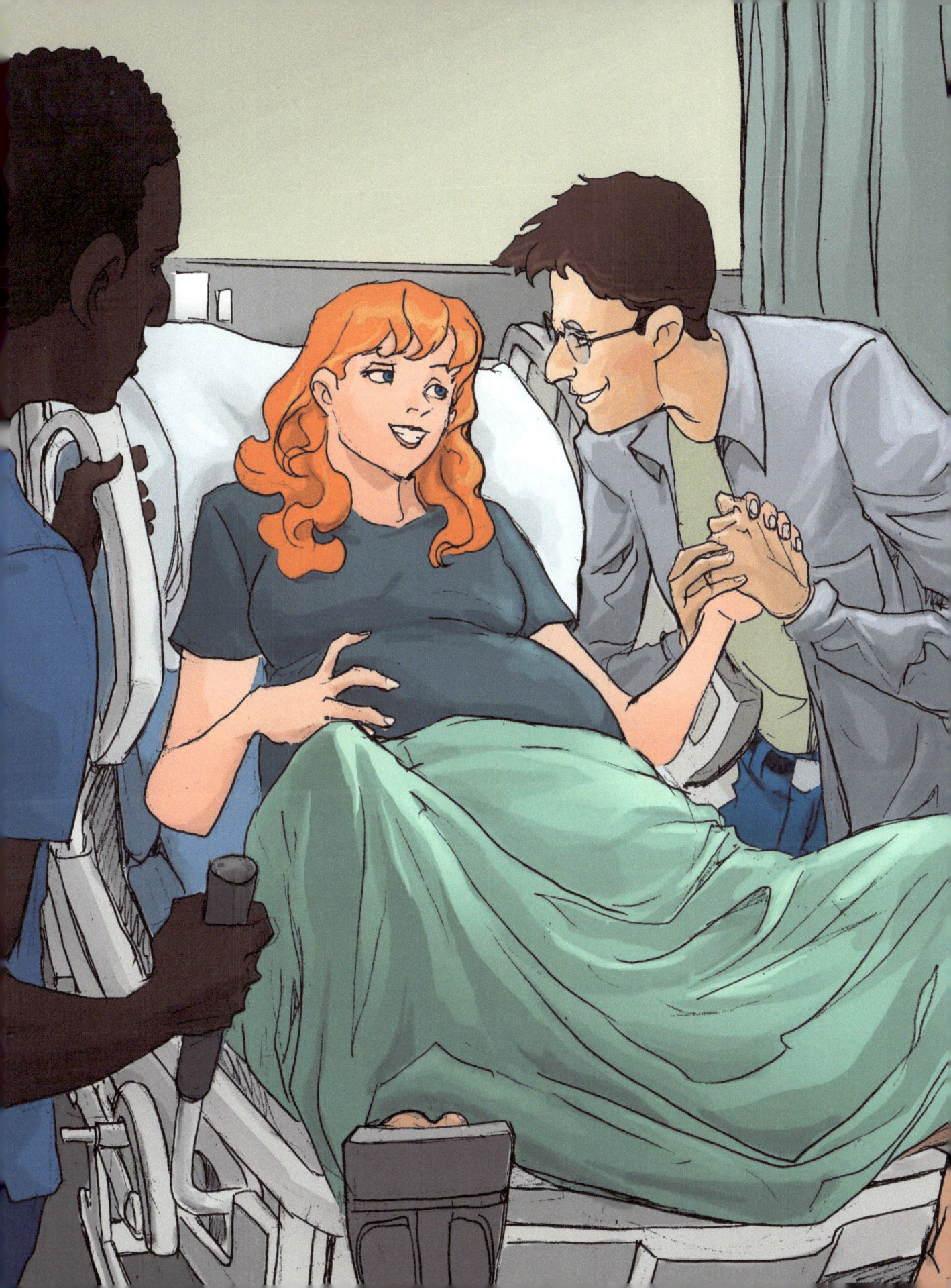

She was born in a
hospital, with the help of
doctors and nurses who
all cared greatly about
her and her mother.
They worked hard
to make sure
that everything went
just right, and it did.

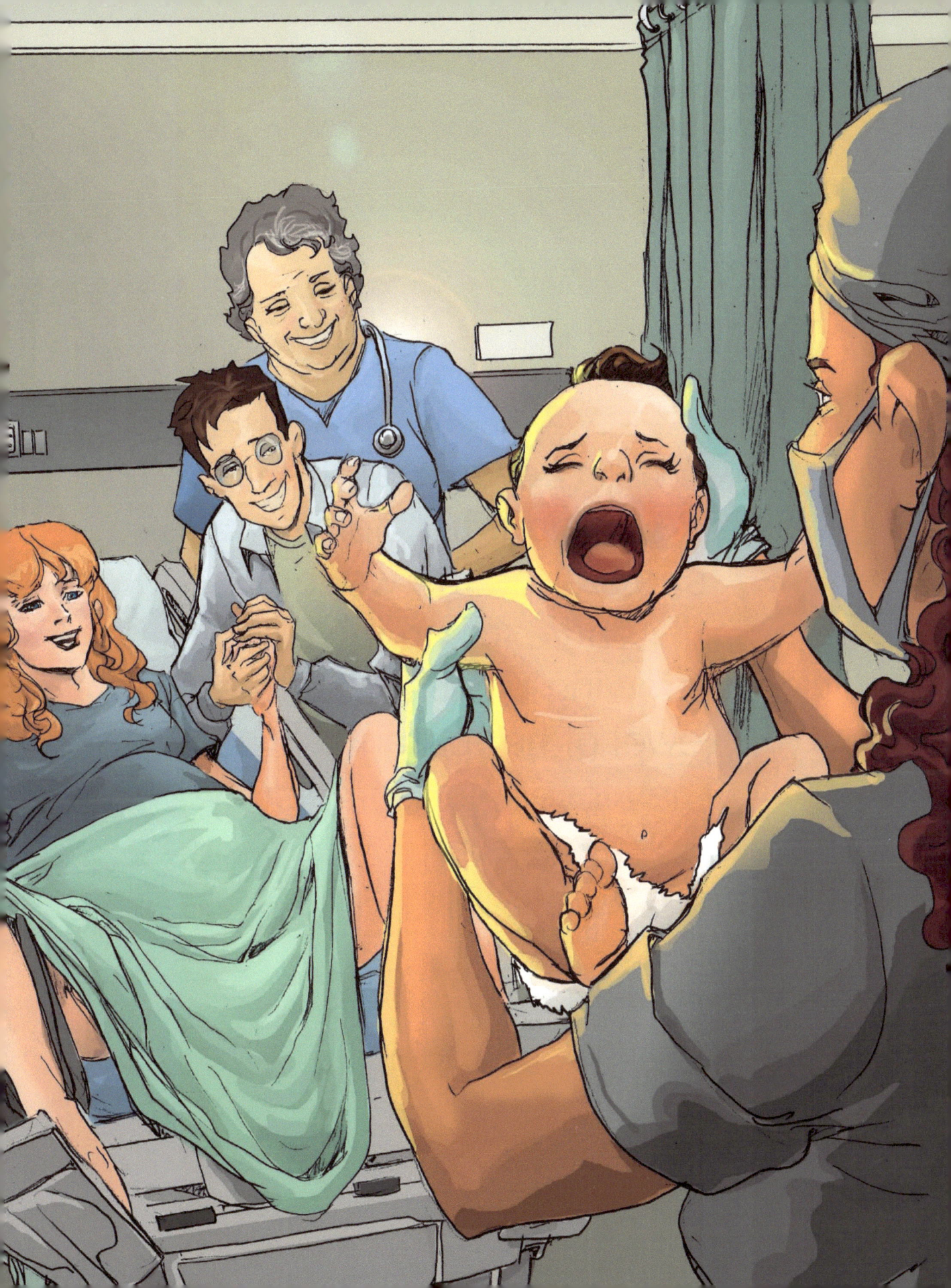

When Jessica's parents
brought her home,
she started the wondrous
and exciting job of
growing up. She was the
jewel of her parents' lives.
They loved her completely!

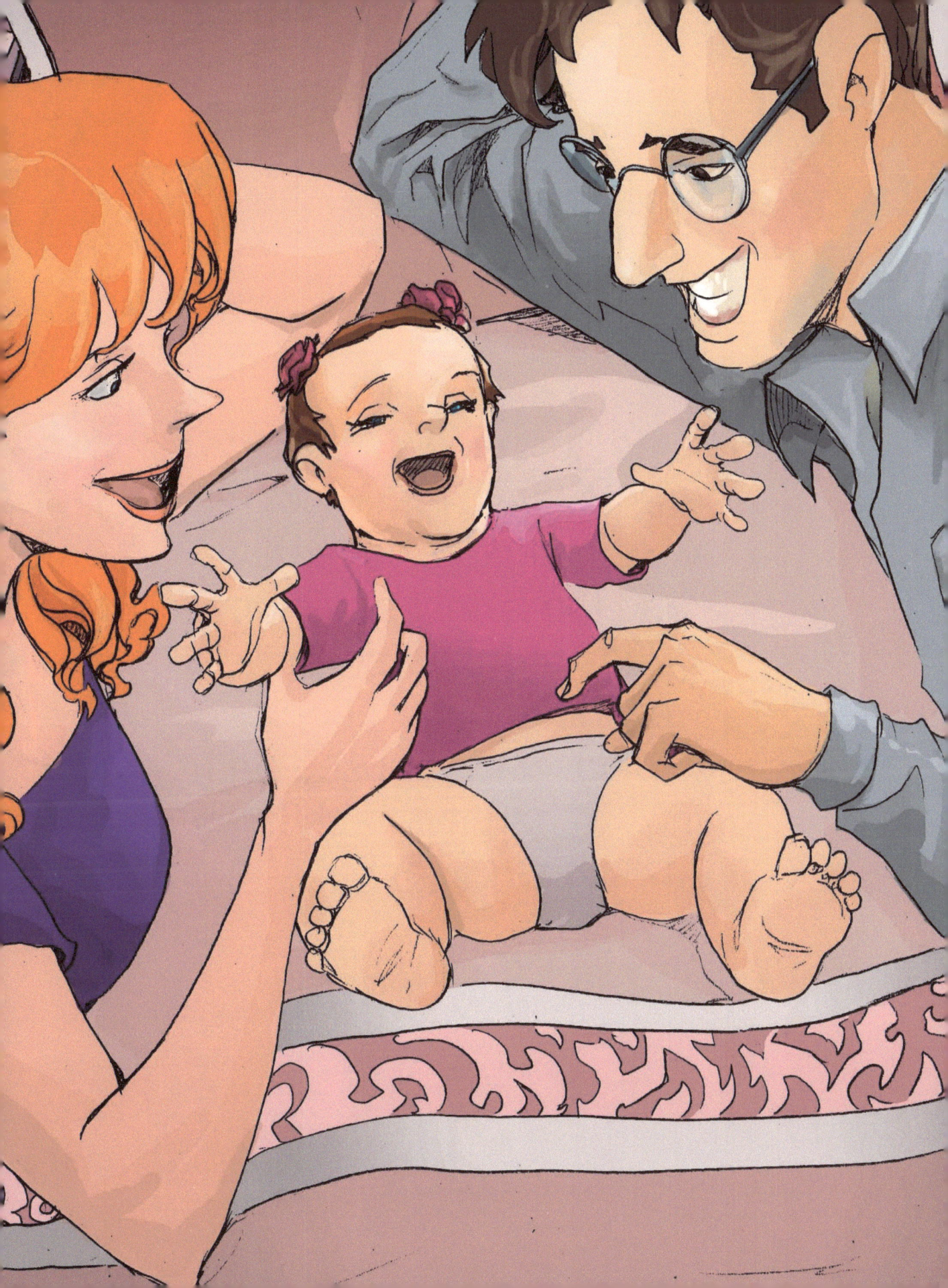

The doctor had told Jessica's parents they should get her vaccinated for her safety and the safety of all the kids around her, but all those other people said vaccines caused bad things to happen to children.

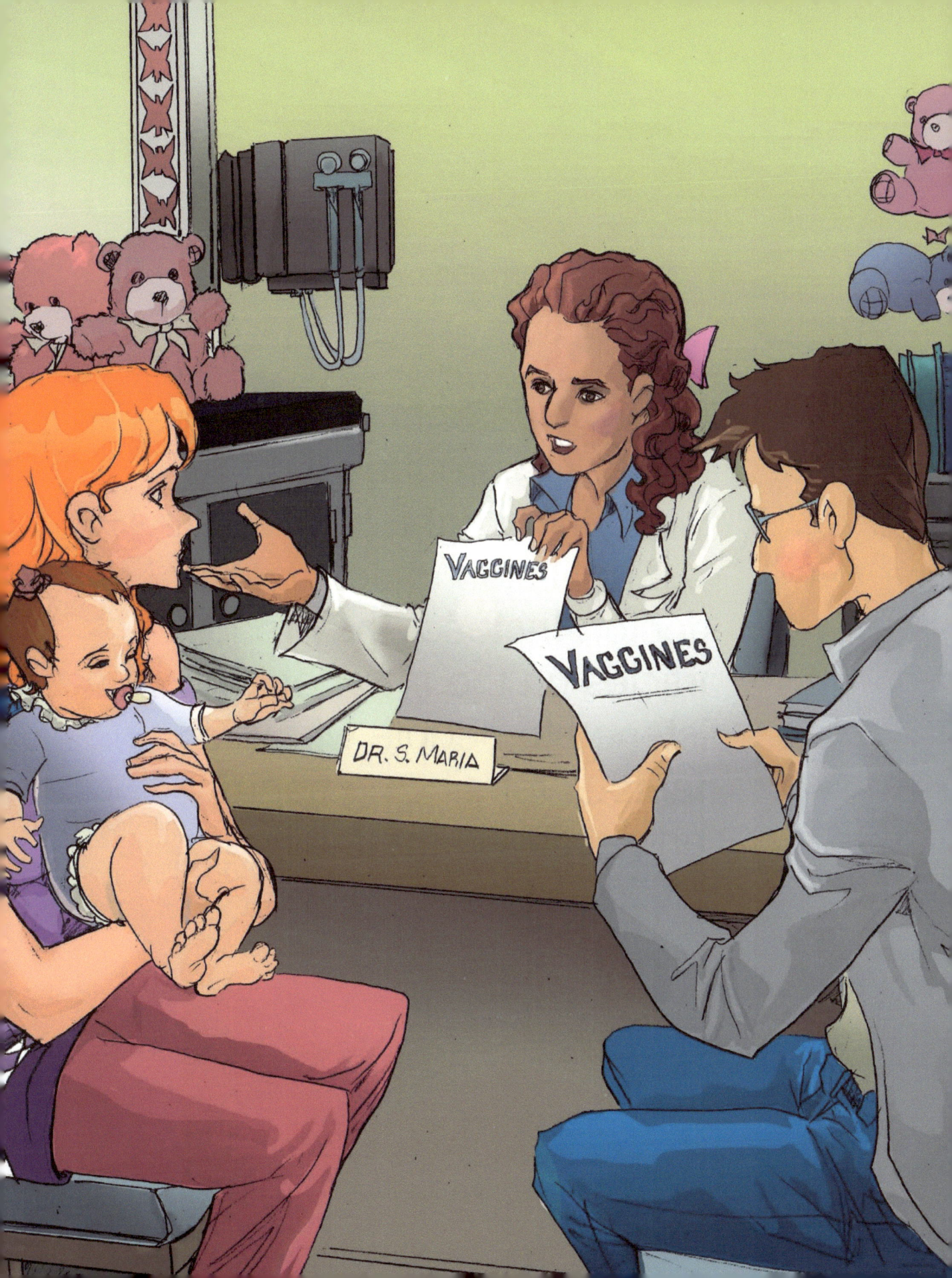

Jessica's parents wanted to make sure they did everything right, but they did not listen to Jessica's doctor. Instead, they read articles on the Internet and listened to people who are famous for singing songs and acting in the movies.

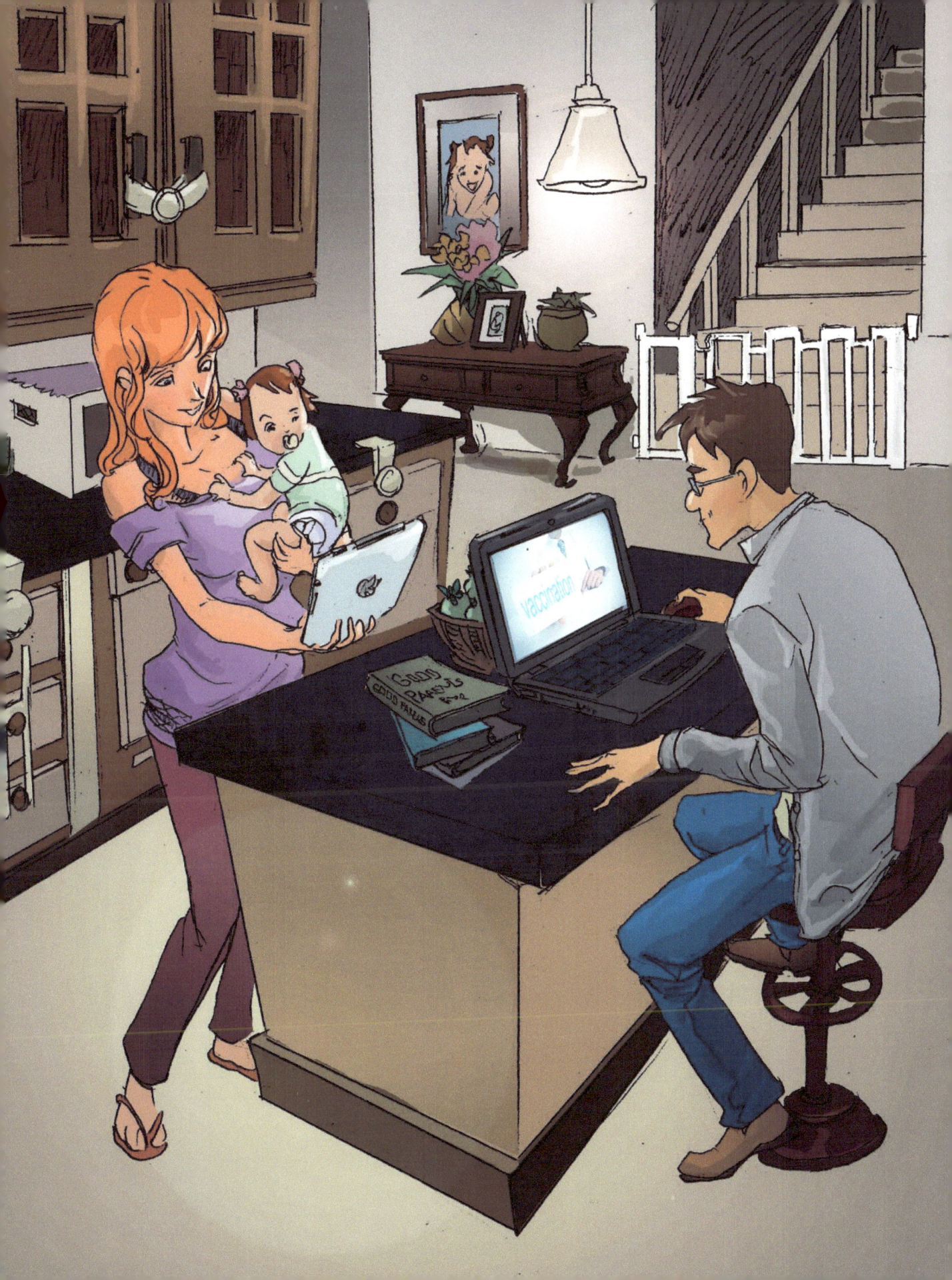

Jessica's parents saw some videos and articles that showed how the claims about bad things happening were wrong, but they ignored them. They trusted and believed the celebrities, because that made them feel good!

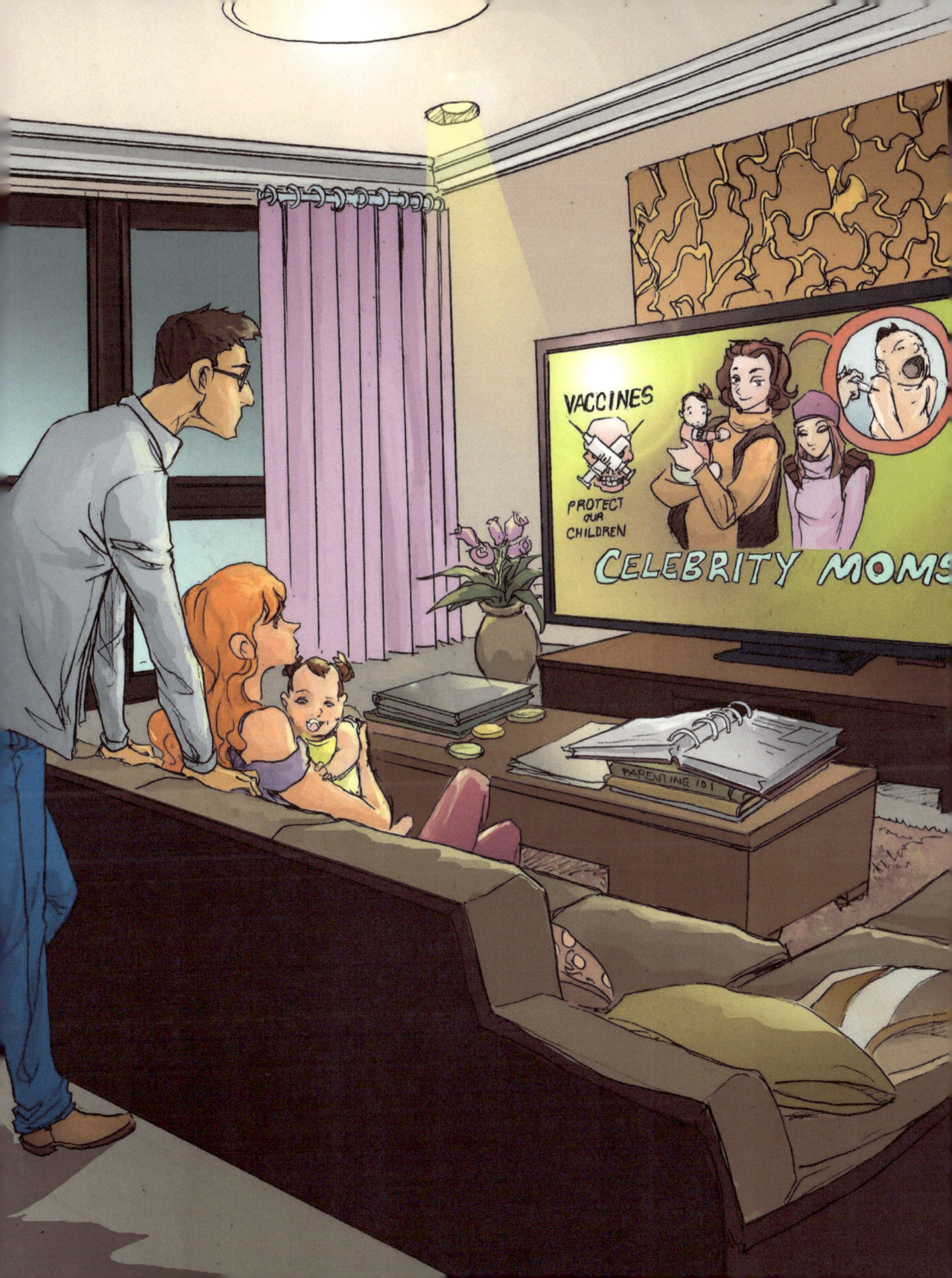

They decided that Jessica should not get vaccines, because so many popular people said vaccines were bad. Jessica's parents didn't stop to think about how they had been vaccinated and were still healthy.

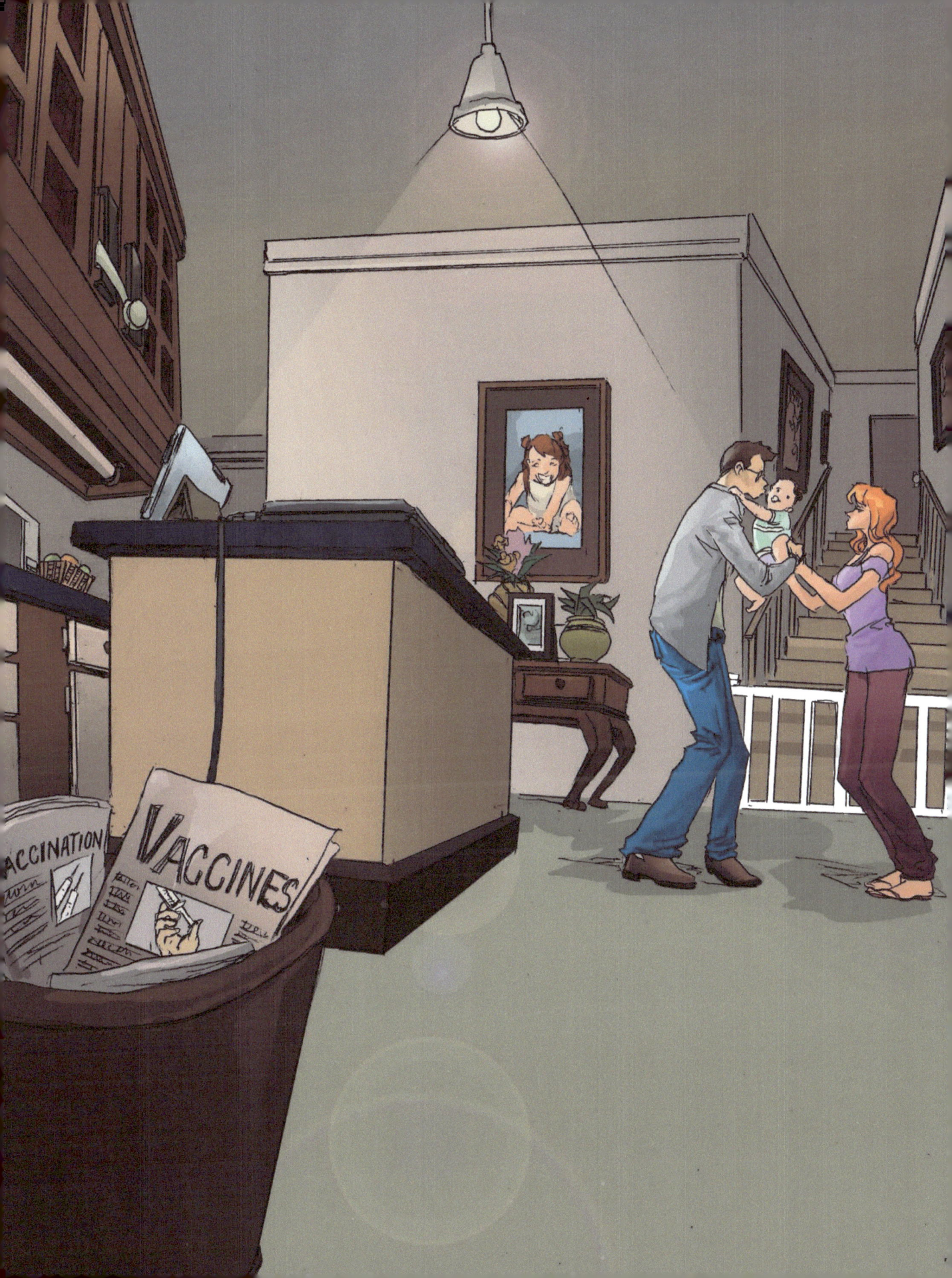

On Jessica's first birthday,
she did not really know
what was going on,
but she had fun
and smiled and laughed.
She was a beautiful and
wonderful baby!

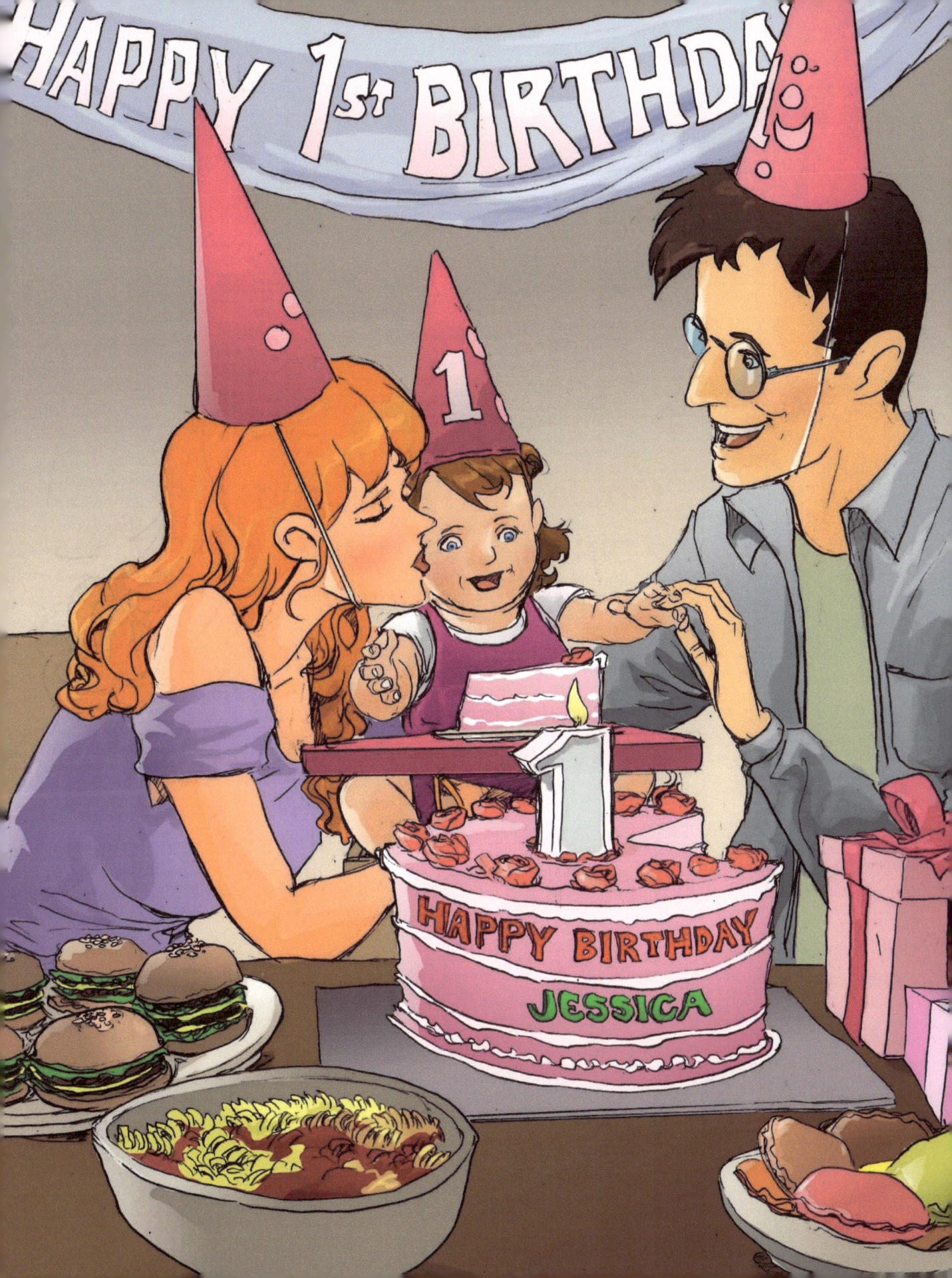

On Jessica's second
birthday, she was
a tiny princess
surrounded by her
princess friends.
It was a fun party!

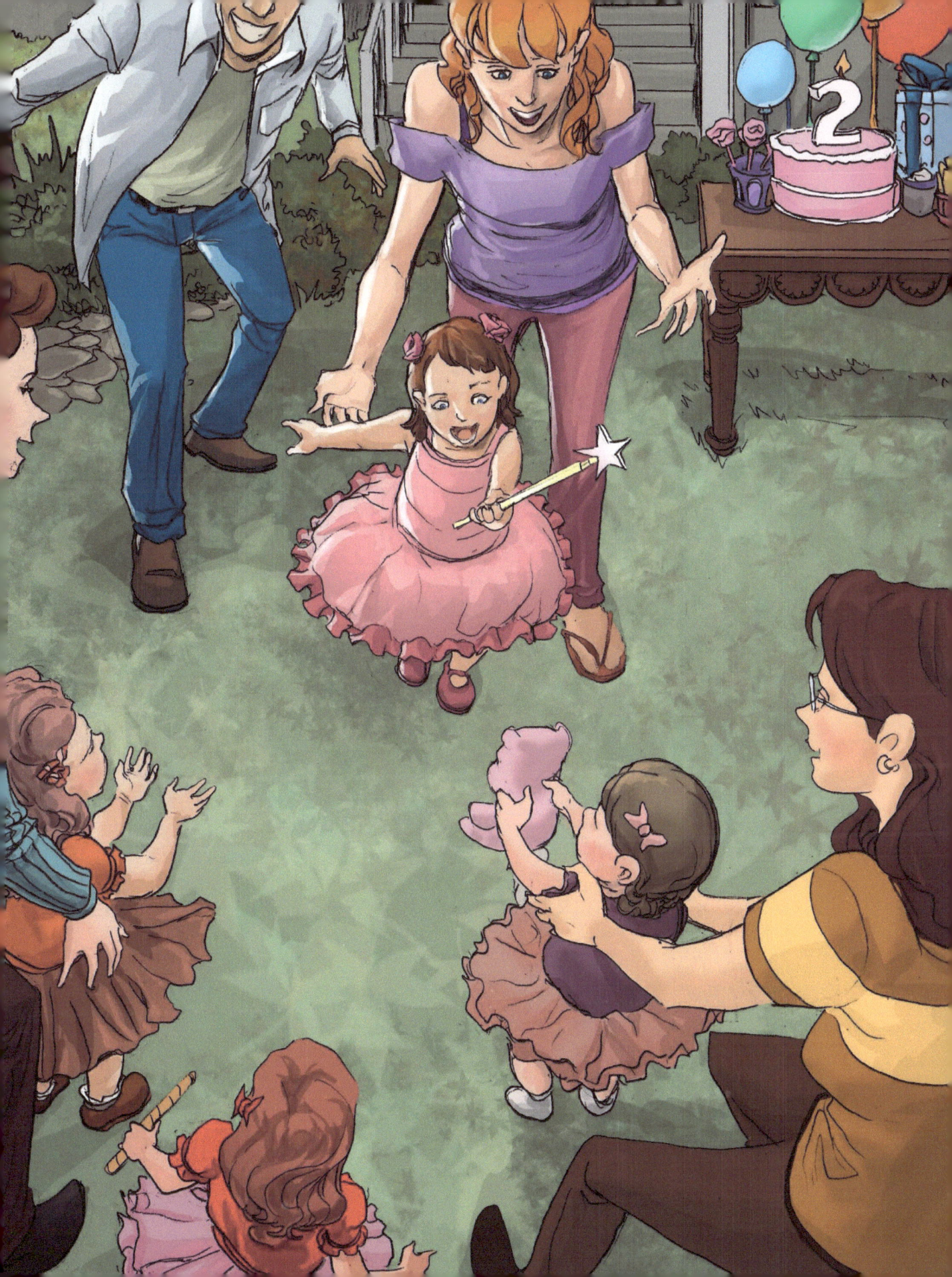

Jessica got measles just
before she turned three.
The doctors and nurses
who helped bring her
into the world tried very
hard to help her,
and Jessica fought
very hard too.

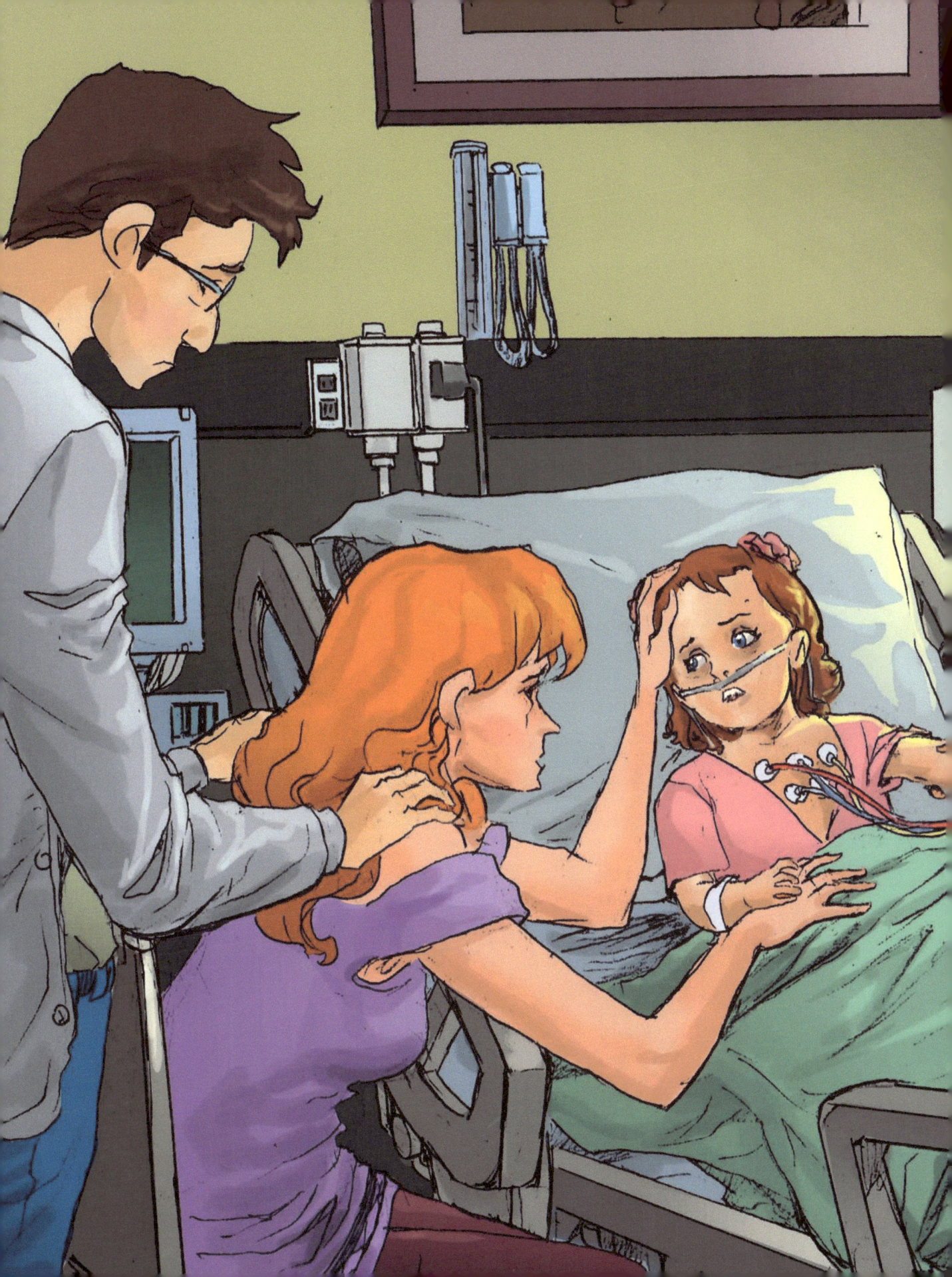

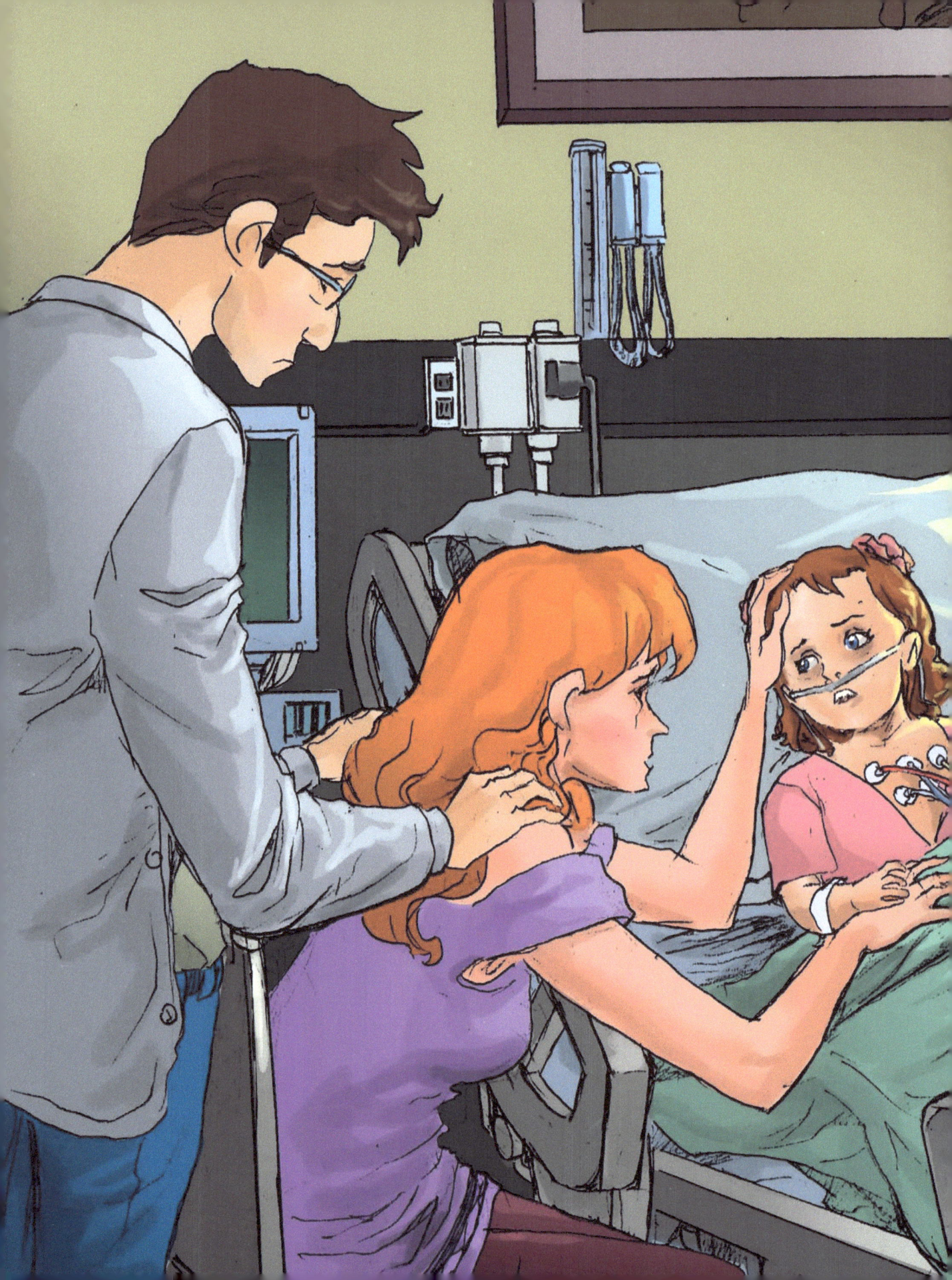

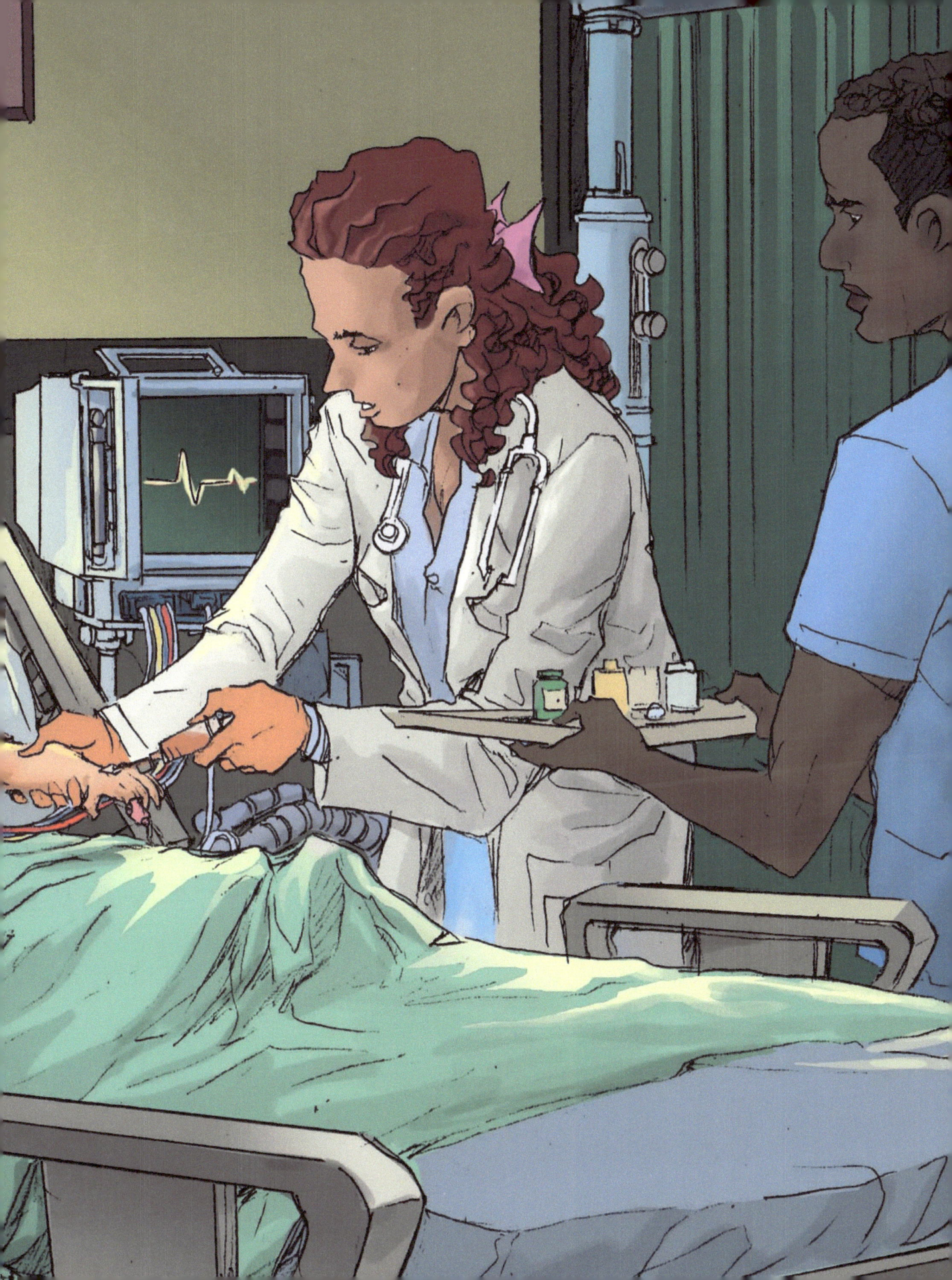

She died –
of complications
from the measles – before
her third birthday.
All because her parents
did a stupid bad thing.
They were sorry they had
made such a terrible mistake,
but it was too late.

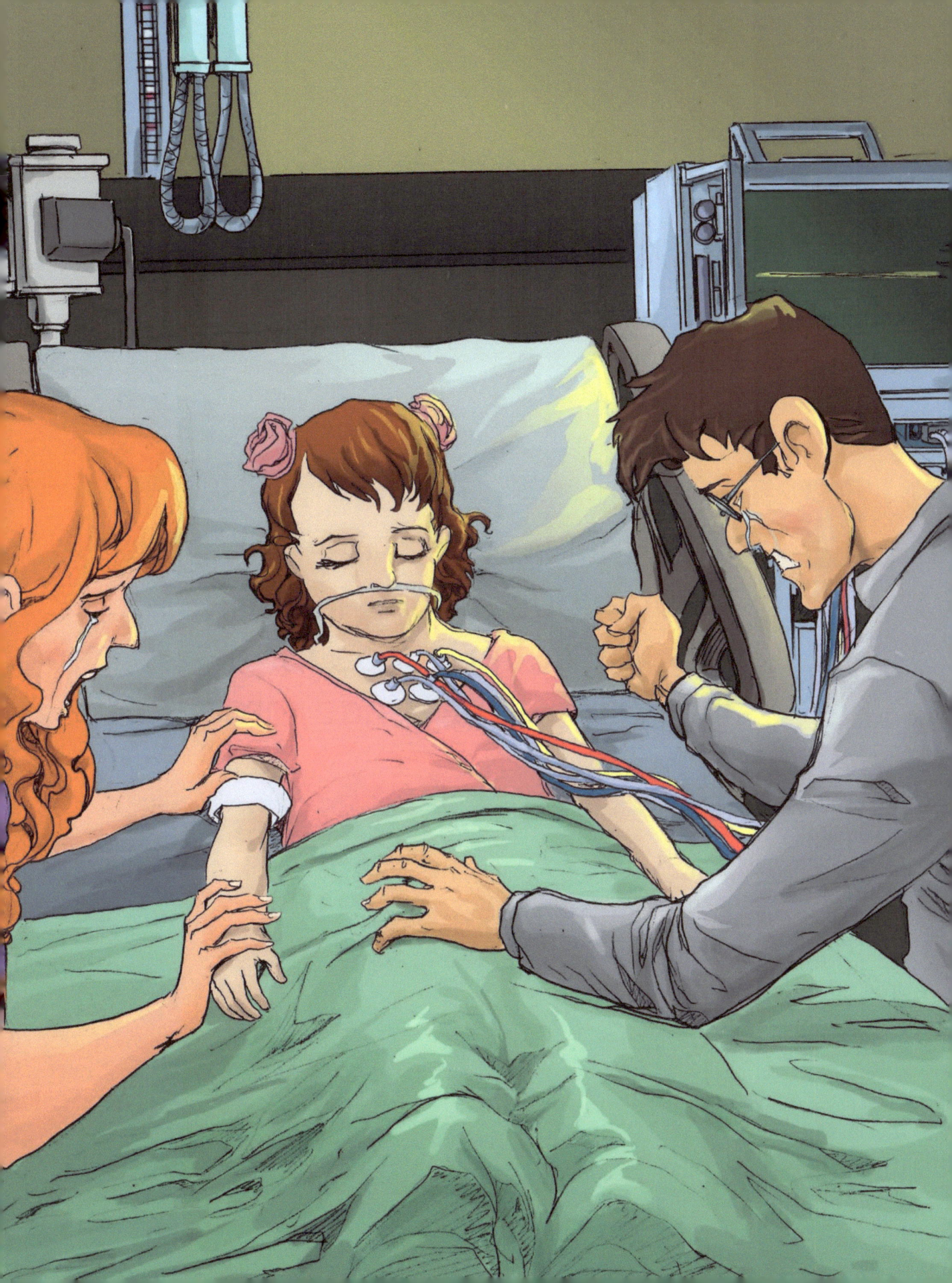

And this is where Jessica's
marvelous story ends – in
a tiny coffin, made for a
little girl – almost age three.

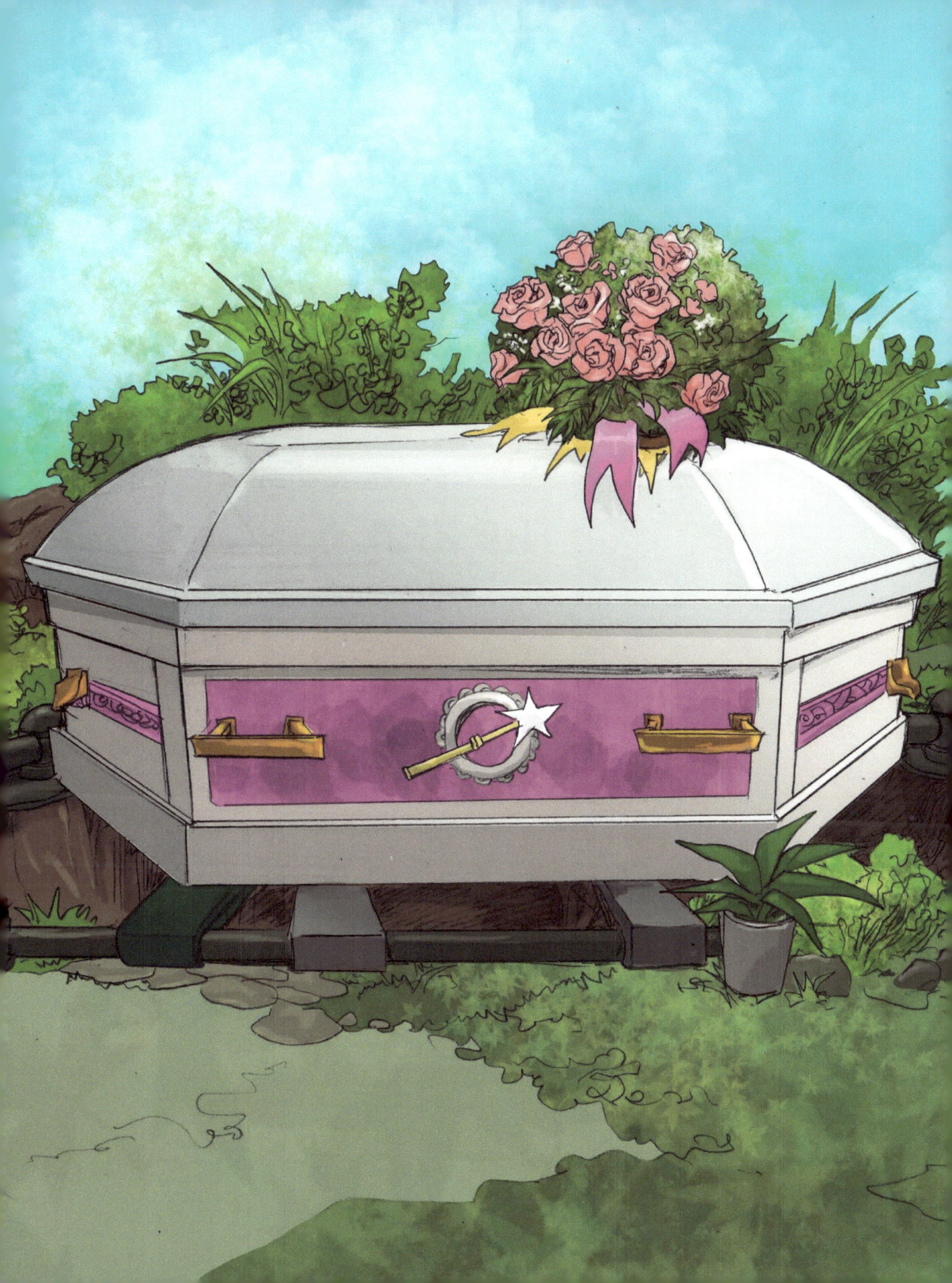

THE END

Stay tuned for:
Carnage at the Kiss-and-Ride
A <u>Not for Kids</u> Tragedy

by Jessica

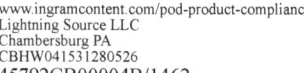